Copyright© 2000, 2004, 2011 by The Dougy Center for Grieving Children. All rights reserved. No part of this publication may be reproduced, stored in a retrieval system, or transmitted in any form or by any means, electronic, mechanical, photocopying, recording or otherwise, without the permission of The Dougy Center, except where short passages are used solely for the purpose of review in television, radio or periodicals.

The Dougy Center for Grieving Children
3909 S.E. 52nd Avenue
P.O. Box 86852 Portland, OR 97286

Phone: 503-775-5683

Fax: 503-777-3097

Email: help@dougy.org

Website: www.dougy.org

Written and printed in the United States of America.

ISBN: 978-1-890534-02-8

Revised 2/2004

Our Mission

The mission of The Dougy Center for Grieving Children is to provide to families in Portland and the surrounding region loving support in a safe place where children, teens and their families grieving a death can share their experiences as they move through their healing process. Through our National Center for Grieving Children & Families we also provide support and training locally, nationally and internationally to individuals and organizations seeking to assist children in grief.

The Dougy Center is supported solely through private support from individuals, foundations and companies, and receives no state or federal funding. The Dougy Center does not charge a fee for its services.

Table of Contents

Development of this guidebook was
made possible through a grant from the
Meyer Memorial Trust

Printing of this guidebook was
made possible through a grant from the
Trust Management Services, LLC.

Introduction

What is it like for teenagers when someone close to them dies? How do they respond to the death of a parent, a sibling, a relative, a friend? In the pages ahead, you'll find practical answers to these questions and information about grief processes as experienced by youth ages 11 to 21. As you read along, you'll notice we use the term "teen" interchangeably with "adolescent" to refer to this age group. We hope that the stories and information presented will assist adults—parents, teachers, youth workers, clergy, relatives— seeking to better understand and improve relationships with grieving teens.

Since its inception in 1982, The Dougy Center for Grieving Children & Families has provided young people with a safe, supportive environment where they can share personal experiences of death and loss. We seek to learn alongside grieving children, teens and their parents or caregivers. They have been our guides and teachers. This guidebook expresses the complexities of the teen grief journey as generously shared with us by hundreds of young people over the years.

In our work with teenagers, we've learned that teens respond to adults who choose to be companions during the grief journey, rather than direct it. We have also discovered that adult companions need to be aware of their own grief issues and journeys, because their experiences and beliefs impact the way they relate to teens.

The words that follow pay tribute to the courageous teens and their adult caregivers who have participated at The Dougy Center over the years. We also salute the dedicated volunteer facilitators at The Dougy Center who invest their time and energy and share their personal grief experiences to provide a safe place for grievers of all ages.

The Grieving Teen

Adolescence is a time of transition between childhood and adulthood. As young teens leave the "child" behind and allow the "teenager" to emerge, they experience anxiety, awkwardness and a sense of loss for the earlier time. With the teenage years come new responsibilities and roles at home and in school. Teens earn a driver's license, take part-time jobs, spend more time with their peers and prepare to leave the nest.

Not surprisingly, the grief journey for a teen is different from that of a child or an adult. The death of a significant person in a teen's life compounds and complicates the developmental process of adolescence. The teenager suddenly finds him or herself dealing with additional issues, including:

- possible unresolved issues with the person who died
- the circumstances of the death
- dramatic changes in his or her life situation
- changes in relationships with others after the death

"In some ways I don't want to grow up. It's sad losing my child identity. I liked being nice and innocent. Now every-thing has to be so adult, so responsible."

—Caleb, 17

The teen's level of emotional and physical maturity, past experiences and family dynamics all influence his or her grief response. Within

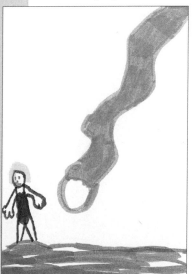

the young griever is a complex mix of emotions, bodily reactions, thoughts, mental pictures, philosophical and religious ideas and behaviors associated with the death.

What Does a Grieving Teen Look Like?

Grieving teens look just like other teens. You won't see them wearing a placard, button or tattoo announcing, "I'm grieving!" You can't pick them out of a crowd of peers because much of their grieving is internal and concealed.

People often confuse "grieving" and "mourning." Grieving refers to the internal experience of the teen, whereas mourning is the public expression of that internal grief. Keep in mind that when a teen loses someone significant, he or she is grieving, whether you can see it or not. Not unlike adults, a teen experiences a broad range of emotions and physical reactions after someone dies. Adults are sometimes surprised to notice that teenagers grieve differently than they do. For example, the death of a close teen friend may evoke more intense grief than the death of a grandparent. Adults who don't expect this can minimize the impact of the peer death because they don't acknowledge or understand the significance of this friendship to the teen.

"My mom couldn't understand how devastated I was when my friend John died in a car accident on his way home from school. She kept saying, 'But you weren't even close friends.' She didn't know how close we were, and I didn't feel like explaining it because she wouldn't understand."

—Kathy, 17

Adolescent Development: Weathering Change and Loss

As many parents know, dealing with teenagers can be challenging under any circumstance. Adolescence is a time of shedding one's identity as a child and assuming the identity of an adult. As teens attain a sense of their own individuality, they rely more on peers and less on parents for support. They also look to their peers for cues on everything from fashion sense to personal values. During this transition, some teens can feel caught between their own desires and the expectations and roles placed on them by the family. For example, teens want to be independent and enjoy their freedom, but depend on their parents for financial support. They also typically wrestle with feelings of competency versus a sense of inadequacy. Adapting to young adulthood and leaving childhood can cause internal conflicts, confusion and even grief. For many teens, and the parents who raise them, the whole experience can be confusing.

Experiencing a death complicates this developmental process. Grieving and mourning, by nature, are characterized by conflicts and paradoxes. For example, grieving teens may feel:

- attached to, yet separated from, the deceased
- ambivalent about the person who died and their previous relationship
- conflicted about letting go of and hanging onto the deceased
- embarrassed about showing emotions
- awkward about being different from their peers

Change, Change, Change

As adolescents are initiated into the adult world, their lives are characterized by a series of changes. Grieving teens undergo the normal range of changes, compounded by the radical shift caused by a death. Adults need to be familiar with developmental changes that occur in adolescence, as well as how those changes are complicated by grief.

Changing bodies are the most obvious change. Teens tend to be extremely concerned about body image and fitting in with their peers. Grieving teens may have a heightened or a diminished interest in physical appearance and peer conformity. Some grieving teens wish they could be children again to avoid growing up and facing increased responsibilities. Some may even regress into more childlike behaviors to meet their emotional needs for nurturance and security.

Changing sexuality is a private matter for teens, seldom discussed with their parents. During childhood, if you have communicated that you are an approachable adult, a teen might seek you out for advice or information about sexuality. Usually, teens have a difficult time discussing their raging hormones with adults—just as they have reservations about discussing their heightened emotions and thoughts about their loss. The confusion of emerging sexuality coupled with major grief reactions is potentially disorienting for teens and parents. Some teens use sexual activity as a diversion from the pain of grief. Like any attempt to run away, this diversion ultimately fails to meet the needs that teens are trying to fulfill.

Changing values often pose conflicts within the family, especially when teens adopt values that are contrary to those of parents or other adults. Issues around money may also present conflicts as adolescents seek more financial freedom and independence. For some teens, sexuality may be expressed in ways adults consider immoral or irresponsible, or which challenge the family's religious beliefs.

Grieving teens may also feel compelled to address meaning-of-life and afterlife issues. Already struggling to find their place in the world, teens in grief may, for a time, experience a crisis of meaning, which adults find perplexing.

"Sometimes I just feel all mixed up, alien, weird."

—Alan, 16

Changing intellectual processes impact grieving teens. While younger children are less able to grasp the finality of death and its consequences, teens may be profoundly aware of the potential consequences of the death. For example, they may internalize comments made about becoming "the man of the house" or "the woman of the house" now that a father or mother has died. They are also aware of the probable financial impacts of the death of a parent. Because teens want to be involved in decision-making and want to know the reasons behind decisions that affect them, conflict may arise as an exhausted, grieving parent attempts to explain or justify his or her decisions.

Changing family relationships often cause anxiety for parents. As the teen increasingly desires to be with peers, he or she may show less interest in family activities, especially if they conflict with peer group events. Parents often feel unappreciated, unloved and unimportant, except as suppliers of trans-portation, money, food and housing. Some parents fight vigorously against these inevitable changes, resulting in increased conflict.

5

Further complicating matters, many parents of grieving teens become overly protective and concerned about the teen's desire to be with peers, forcing a conflict between the teen's desire for independence and the parents' wishes for security and control. Grieving teens need the stability, consistency and safety created by loving adults. However, they are not well served by overprotectiveness and resistance to their natural maturing processes.

The combination of adolescent development and grieving increases the potential for negative responses from the teen. Accepting, attentive adults who have come to terms with their own grief journeys can help to significantly reduce the potential of detrimental outcomes for grieving teens. Adults need to remember that the grieving teen:

- was a child not long ago

- possesses few resources for grieving

- has little experience dealing with death and grieving

- inhabits an almost-adult body, but often feels like a child

- may be trying to cope with a grieving parent(s), sibling, family member, friend, etc.

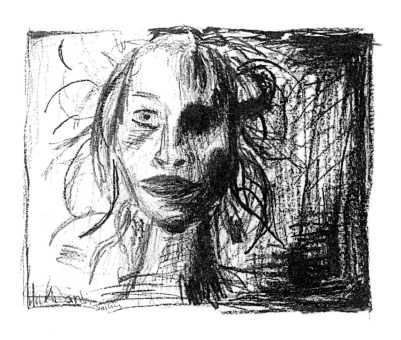

Six Basic Principles of Teen Grief

1. Grieving is the teen's natural reaction to a death.

Grief is a natural reaction to death and other losses. However, grieving does not feel natural because it can be difficult to control emotions, thoughts or physical feelings associated with a death. The sense of being out of control, that is often a part of grief, may overwhelm or frighten some teens. Grieving is normal and healthy, yet may be an experience teens resist and reject. Helping teens accept the reality that they are grievers allows them to do their grief work and progress in their grief journey.

"I hate it when people think I should be grieving according to the stages described in some high school health book. Since my sister's death, I've learned that grief isn't five simple stages."

—*Kimberly, 17*

2. Each teen's grieving experience is unique.

Grieving is a different experience for each person. Teens grieve for different lengths of time and express a wide spectrum of emotions. Grief is best understood as a process in which bodily sensations, emotions, thoughts and behaviors surface in response to the death, its circumstances, the past relationship with the deceased and the realization of the future without the person. For example, sadness and crying may be an expression of grief for one teen, while another may respond with humor and laughter.

While many theories and models of the grieving process provide a helpful framework, the path itself is individual, and often lonely. No book or grief therapist can predict or prescribe exactly what a teen will or should go through on the grief journey. Adults can best assist grieving teenagers by accompanying them on their journey in the role of listener and learner, and by allowing the teen to function as a teacher.

3. There are no "right" and "wrong" ways to grieve.

Sometimes, adults express strong opinions about "right" or "wrong" ways to grieve. But there is no correct way to grieve. Coping with a death does not follow a simple pattern or set of rules, nor is it a course to be evaluated or graded.

There are, however, "helpful" and "unhelpful" choices and behaviors associated with the grieving process. Some behaviors are constructive and encourage facing grief, such as talking with trusted friends, journaling, creating art and expressing emotion, rather than holding it inside. Other grief responses are destructive and can cause long-term complications and consequences. For example, some teens attempt to escape their pain through many of the same escape routes adults choose: alcohol and substance abuse, reckless sexual activity, antisocial behaviors, withdrawal from social activities, excessive sleeping, high risk-taking behaviors, and other methods that temporarily numb the pain of their loss.

"My friend went crazy into drugs, sex, and skipping school after her boyfriend got killed in a skiing accident. She stopped talking about him. Now she's kicked out of school and is pregnant by a guy she hates. Since my boyfriend's car accident, I know what can happen if I make wrong choices like her."

—*Sara, 18*

4. Every death is unique and is experienced differently.

The way teens grieve differs according to their personality and the particular relationship they had with the deceased. They typically react in different ways to the death of a parent, sibling, grandparent, child or friend. For many teens, peer relationships are primary. The death or loss of a boyfriend or girlfriend may seem to affect them more than the death of a sibling or grandparent.

Within a family, each person may mourn differently at different times. One may be talkative, another may tend to cry often, and a third might withdraw. This can generate a great deal of tension and misunderstanding within the already-stressed family. Each person's responses to death should be honored as his or her way of coping in that moment. Keep in mind that responses may change from day to day or even hour to hour.

"Expect the unexpected. Emily actually danced and sang after I told her that her mother died. I was shocked. Later I realized the relief we both felt. The relationship had been filled with her alcoholism, lies and illness."

—*Father of Emily, 17*

5. The grieving process is influenced by many issues.

The impact of a death on a teen relates to a combination of factors, including:

- social support systems available for the teen (family, friends and/or community)
- circumstances of the death; how, where and when the person died
- whether the young person unexpectedly found the body
- the nature of the relationship with the person who died—harmonious, abusive, conflictual, unfinished, communicative
- the teen's level of involvement in the dying process
- the emotional and developmental age of the teen
- the teen's previous experiences with death

6. Grief is ongoing.

Grief never ends, but it does change in character and intensity. Many grievers have compared their grieving to the constantly shifting tides of the ocean; ranging from calm, low tides to raging high tides that change with the seasons and the years.

The "never-ending, but changing" aspect of grief may be one of the least understood. Most people are anxious for teens to have closure and "put the death behind them" so they can move on. But death leaves a vacuum in the lives of those left behind. Life is never the same again. This does not mean that life can never be joyful again, nor that the experience of loss cannot be transformed into something positive. But grief does not have a magical closure. People report pangs of grief 40, 50, even 60 years after a death. Grief is not a disease that can be cured, but rather a process we
learn to incorporate into our lives.

> *"I've had people say that you've got to go on, you've got to get over this. I just want to shout, 'You're wrong! Grief never ends.' I don't care what they say."*
>
> *—Philip, 13*

Emotions and the Grieving Teen

Teens may experience a wide range of emotions after the loss of someone significant in their lives. Even so, they may exhibit few outward signs of grief. Some young people find it difficult to express emotions, particularly sadness for boys and anger for girls.

When they feel vulnerable, teens may resist sharing because it magnifies their feelings around the loss. They fear that if they allow themselves to feel the pain, it will overwhelm them.

Here are some common words that teens at The Dougy Center have used to describe how they feel:

disbelief • shock • astonishment • alone • alarm

awkward • embarrassed • tense • fearful • scared

irritated • angry • envious • jealous • numb • cold

frigid • weird • apprehensive • isolated • lonely

powerless • confused • frustrated • ambivalent • eager

relieved • hopeful • out-of-control • assured • happy

glad • renewed • energetic • tired • positive • shallow

unorganized • stupid • goal-less • meaningless

resentful • strange • outraged • revengeful

Anger

Anger is a normal emotion for grievers of all ages. Teens commonly feel and express anger after a death. In part, they feel angry because it seems unfair that they should have to suffer the death of someone in their lives, especially at such an early age. Teens may also be angry at specific people—the deceased, themselves, the police, parents and/or medical professionals. Or, they may be angry at God, fate or the entire world.

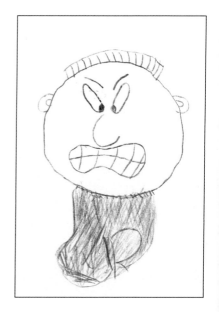

Frustration

Frustration often resembles anger because it is expressed in a similar fashion. People feel frustrated when they cannot meet goals, intentions or expectations. Grieving teens are frustrated because their world has changed so drastically and unexpectedly. Goals they previously had in the areas of relationships, academic pursuits and financial stability appear unattainable in the face of the death and its accompanying changes. Frustration can arise when:

- the teen did not get to say goodbye
- there is unfinished business between the teen and the deceased
- financial problems arise
- a parent becomes overprotective
- grades decline because of difficulties focusing
- the teen is not told the truth about the death
- peers tease or make fun of the teen
- questions about a death go unanswered
- a perpetrator is not apprehended
- a body cannot be located, or a death cannot be verified

Helpful Hints for Anger and Frustration

Angry teens who act out with destructive behavior have difficulty hearing the concerns of adults. Frequently, adults respond to anger by telling teens they shouldn't *feel* a certain way, while demanding that they stop the behavior. Failing to validate the teen's anger tends to fuel it. A better approach is to help teens find safe ways to express anger without hurting themselves or others. Some safe outlets for teens to expend energy and constructively cope with anger include:

- participating in sports or athletic activities
- boxing a punching bag or pounding on a pillow
- using the body's big muscles through sports or exercise
- expressing feelings and thoughts through creative writing and art
- yelling or screaming in a safe place
- sculpting with clay or Play-Doh

For teens who experience the frustration of failing to meet goals and expectations, breaking down tasks into manageable steps is often helpful. Sometimes, doing homework with a friend is helpful. Parents can assist in this process by offering guidance in problem solving and goal setting.

Anxiety

Feeling anxious, worried and off-balance is a typical response to a death because of the drastic changes in relationships and circumstances associated with the experience. Some teens may even develop panic attacks. Signs of a panic attack include:

- palpitating heartbeat
- difficulty breathing
- throbbing in the head or neck
- dizziness, or a sense of feeling paralyzed

Helpful Hints about Anxiety

Mild feelings of anxiety are not a cause for concern. However, persistent symptoms of anxiety, panic attacks or dramatic changes in mood should be checked by a medical professional. To help teens coping with mild anxiety, you might encourage relaxing activities, such as deep breathing, yoga, listening to soothing music or meditation.

Guilt

After her father's death from a heart attack, Kim, age 17, was tormented by the thought that she might have saved her father's life. "I just played around when we were practicing CPR in health class. If I had learned it better, maybe I could have saved my dad. I should have been able to do it better. I was scared and forgot everything." When her mother learned of Kim's self-blame, she encouraged Kim to read the coroner's report. Reading the facts helped Kim understand that even a skilled EMT or coronary physician could not have saved her father because of the condition of his heart. Later she reported, "I felt so relieved after feeling so guilty for so long. I wish I had talked to my mom earlier. But I thought she wouldn't understand. I thought she blamed me, too."

"I should have stopped Scott from driving after the party. I knew he was mad at me. He was always fighting with me over drinking and driving too fast. I kept telling him he'd get in an accident. I tried to stop him from leaving but ... Now I have to be mad at him for dying in that stupid car."

—Mindy, 18

Helpful Hints about Guilt

Many teens believe that they could or should have done something to prevent the death. Attempting to convince the teen that it was not his or her fault usually doesn't alleviate guilt. Instead, allowing the teen to process what he or she thinks and feels about the death will gradually help reduce the self-blame and guilt. Often, a teen feels guilty because he or she did not do more before the death, and believes that the person who died could or should have received more attention. Survivors of a suicide often feel at fault for missing warning clues, not recognizing 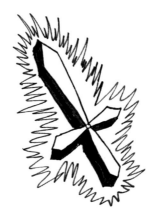 plans that led to the death or allowing lethal weapons or medications in the house.

Arguing that the teen was not to blame does not assist the griever and can pressure the teen to bury the guilt and grief. If a teen feels responsible or blames him or herself, here are some ways you can help:

- Listen and restate what you heard in your own words so he or she feels heard and understood.

- Ask questions to help the teen work through the grief:

    "What do you wish you had done?"

    "Explain to me what you think you did wrong."

    "How do you think you could have changed the outcome?"

    "What is it you think you could have done, or should have done differently?"

    "What's the hardest part about this for you?"

    "What do you think [the deceased] would want you to do?"

- Avoid "why?" questions, which usually fuel conflict and may cause defensive reactions.

- Explain the facts about the cause of death.

- Allow the teen to voice his or her feelings without fixing or judging.

As difficult as it can be to listen to teens blame themselves, it is usually more helpful to explore their feelings further by asking questions and expressing concern, rather than telling them that what they're feeling is not true.

When a teen bears some responsibility for the death

Sometimes a teen has played some part in the death. In these situations, he or she needs to feel and work through guilt and regrets. Attempting to dissuade the teen from feeling guilt or minimizing the responsibility may complicate, rather than alleviate, the grief process. Helping the young person face that area of responsibility and discover options for acknowledging the guilt and making restitution can facilitate healing. Some actions that can speed healing and result in significant maturing for a teen in this situation include:

- seeking forgiveness
- making restitution where possible
- accepting the legal punishment when ordered

Isolation

Many teens feel isolated from their friends after a death. They often say that no one understands what they are going through. Typically, teens may be aware that there are other people their own age who have experienced similar deaths but are not connected with them. Because of this, they feel misunderstood and alone.

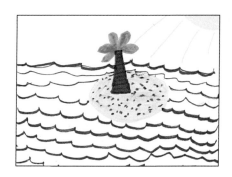

Helpful Hints about Isolation

Finding peers who have also experienced a death can be quite helpful to the grieving adolescent. Teens can learn about peer experiences of loss through support groups, books, movies and counseling sessions. Connecting with others alleviates feelings of isolation and may provide a supportive network in which teens can address ongoing feelings and concerns.

Relief

It is not uncommon for teens who experience the death of a chronically ill person or of an abusive person to feel a sense of relief. Feelings of relief are partly due to the reality that the painful, uncomfortable or embarrassing aspects of the person's experience or actions have ended.

"I was relieved when my mom finally died. She had been in so much pain. It was hard to see her suffer."

—*D'Shanna, 14*

Helpful Hints about Responding to Relief

As with anger and other emotions surrounding grief, it is important to validate rather than dismiss relief. Otherwise, teens may feel guilty, disapproved of and misunderstood. One way to do this is to normalize the experience of relief by discussing situations in which relief was a natural reaction.

Revenge and Rage

In some cases, due to the circumstances and cause of death, teens may experience strong emotions such as revenge and rage. These reactions may be directed against the perpetrator, the deceased or others.
A death that seems vicious and unjustifiable provokes emotional responses of revenge and rage against anyone who contributed to the death or the troubling consequences that followed. Circumstances of death that evoke such strong emotions may include suicide and murder, as well as situations where teens feel the deceased somehow contributed to his or her death, such as not taking needed medication, smoking, drinking or failing to seek medical help in time.

Helpful Hints about Handling Rage

Help your teens discuss strong emotions while encouraging them toward healthy behaviors to release anger and relax. Counseling and support groups may also be appropriate arenas to work through powerful emotions such as rage.

Sadness

Most teens feel melancholy and "blue" after a death. This is a natural response to a person being gone and the inevitable life changes brought about by their loss. Sometimes the sadness will last a long time. Occasionally, teens identify so closely with the person who died that they believe they would be disloyal to feel anything other than unhappiness. They equate love and respect for the deceased person with feeling and acting sad. This may be because someone has taught them, directly or indirectly, that love and loyalty to the dead are expressed by degrees of sadness. Also, teens may fear that letting go of intense sadness means they're forgetting the person who died.

"Sometimes I feel like I'm in this great big, black tunnel; the walls are slimy and I can't climb out. I claw my way up; then I slip back. Deeper and deeper I seem to sink."

—*John, 17*

Helpful Hints about Sadness

Because this may be their first experience with the death of a close person, teens may need reassurance that love for the deceased can be expressed through other emotions. Feeling joy and happiness about life events need not be perceived as betrayal of the person who died.

Sadness and prolonged, chronic depression are very different things. When a teen shows long-lasting withdrawal, lack of energy and motivation, he or she should have a mental health evaluation. Any signs or talk about suicide, wishing to die or joining the deceased should be taken seriously and the teen evaluated by a professional. It is not unusual for teens to express such feelings following a significant loss, but most teens who attempt or complete suicide have shown signs and even discussed their intentions with others.

"This grief stuff feels like I'm caught in a big spider web and this huge spider is about to suck the life out of me."

—*Ryan, 14*

14 Ways to Assist Grieving Teens

1. Listen, care for and accept teens as they are

2. Tell the truth and answer their questions honestly

3. Encourage them to make healthy and creative choices in dealing with their pain and healing process

4. Invite them to view the body, participate in the memorial and burial or see the cremated remains

5. Suggest they create memory rituals, talk about the person and recall memories

6. Discuss their perceptions, experiences and beliefs

7. Acknowledge their loss of focus and interest

8. Be steady and stable during this turbulent period

9. Seek help for your own grief process through appropriate means such as peers, support groups or a professional therapist

10. Affirm and appreciate your children during this difficult time

11. Assure the adolescent of your love and respect

12. Use words and expressions of comfort and affection

13. Express that you appreciate and value the uniqueness and differences between the siblings

14. Accept each teen's unique grief process

Common Reactions to Loss

Grief is expressed in many different behaviors. Often people expect to see grief expressed in just a few ways: crying, sad facial expressions, inactivity or talking about the person who died and the circumstances of the death. Grieving may include but is not limited to these behaviors.

Academic Problems

Grieving teens commonly experience general academic problems, such as lower test scores and grades, poor work habits and truancy. They may expend considerable mental energy in their attempts to make sense of the whole experience surrounding death, leaving little in reserve for academic pursuits and assignments. Teen grievers often find themselves staring into space or daydreaming, unable to focus on a lecture or assignment.

Helpful Hints about Academic Problems

If school assignments can be modified to allow grieving students to channel their emotions and energy into writing, drawing or other school projects, teens may not fall as far behind in school while they also work through their grief. It is often helpful if parents and teachers talk about the teen's grief and work together to lessen the work assignments, then assign a buddy, who will help the teen with assignments, or a tutor, who will be able to work individually with the teen.

Crying

Crying is one of many ways to express grief. Teens may tear up, but not cry. It should not be assumed that a teen must or should cry while grieving, or that they aren't grieving because they're not crying.

Crying publicly can be a beneficial release of feelings for some, but many young people choose to cry only in the privacy of their own rooms or other safe places, or only when alone.

Some teens have little experience with crying and worry about being consumed by it. Therefore, they refuse to start. Fear of embarrassment and vulnerability stifles tears. They may fear that if they let themselves feel the pain, the grief will be overwhelming.

"I haven't even told my friends how I feel. I just smile or make everybody laugh so they don't know how much it hurts. I don't talk to my mom because I don't want her to feel worse. When I talked to her, she got all teary. I felt like crying, too. No way am I going to cry."

—Randy, 14

Helpful Hints about Crying

Creating a safe, nonjudgmental atmosphere tends to allow young people to express their grief by crying, if that seems beneficial to them. Allowing teens to grieve with or without tears accommodates their unique grieving process.

Eating Problems and Disorders

For some teens, grief is expressed primarily through the body. Indigestion, flatulence, nausea and constipation may persist for some grievers. For teens, eating problems associated with grief can develop into more serious eating disorders, such as bulimia and anorexia—particularly prevalent among girls. Girls are especially susceptible to eating disorders because of the pressures to be thin and emphasis on physical appearance in our culture.

These secretive ways of coping with difficult feelings—by binge eating and purging—often go unnoticed by adults. Pushing food away becomes a way to push pain away. Bulimia numbs the body; purging is often an attempt to regain control. A family's unwillingness to talk about the death might block healthy grief outlets and contribute to eating problems and disorders as a coping mechanism of an adolescent.

Helpful Hints about Eating Problems

Parents of grieving teens need to notice changes in appetite and be attentive to unusual behaviors related to food, such as:

- unwillingness to eat

- disappearance of certain foods, secretive eating

- withdrawal at meal times

- bloodshot eyes

- vomiting sounds, vomit odors in the bathroom

- preoccupation with conversations about feeling fat or wishing to lose weight

- thinning of the cheeks

Adults who see any disturbing signs are urged to contact a medical doctor or counselor. Eating disorders can be life-threatening.

Nightmares and Dreams

Nightmares and dreams about the deceased are typical after a loss. These dreams may be comforting, disturbing, inspirational or frightening. Vivid dreams, visitations and other sleep-related phenomenon are common for grieving people of all ages. Many teens report remembering detailed, troubling dreams or humorous encounters with the deceased.

Nightmares cause difficulties for teens, not only because of their potentially terrifying emotional content, but also because they frequently disturb sleep patterns, resulting in increased fatigue and irritability.

"In the dream, my dad was sitting at the head of the table reading his morning newspaper where he always sat. I was eating my favorite cereal. He stopped reading and put his newspaper down. He said, 'Megan, it is time for you to move on; it's been almost two years.' I stared at him and said, 'Dad, this is not like plastic surgery. I'll move on when I want to.' "

—Megan, 18

Helpful Hints about Nightmares

A parent who wishes to help a teen bothered by nightmares might ask:

- Would you like me to leave you alone, or come sit with you?
- Would you like your light on or off?
- Do you want me to hold you, or not touch you?
- Do you want to tell me about your nightmare or not?

"Sometimes I dream my dad is back. He's alive; we're really doing some fun things and laughing. It's just like old times. Then I wake up. I'm feeling really, really good. But then it hits me: he is dead. He's never coming back. A black cloud seems to drift over me. I feel really, really heavy."

—*David, 16*

Listen to your teen talk about the nightmare. Do not judge or explain what you think it means (unless you're asked to), and resist the temptation to try to "make it better" by making it go away. Powerful information and healing can result from teens processing their dreams and nightmares. Reassure your teen that nightmares and dreams about the deceased are normal, common reactions to grieving. If nightmares or other sleep disturbances persist and disrupt your teen's daily functioning, professional evaluation may be needed.

Physical Reactions

Grieving includes all sorts of feelings and physical responses for teens. Many grievers have prolonged physical changes or reactions to loss, including:

- weight loss or gain
- headaches or migraines
- anxiety/panic attacks
- insomnia, fatigue, lethargy; sleeping more than usual
- internal pain, muscle aches
- digestive problems
- heavy breathing, palpitating heartbeat, throbbing

- dizziness or disequilibrium
- visual impairment
- problems with urination, constipation
- dehydration or dry mouth, congestion
- increased susceptibility to illnesses and infections

When experienced in moderation, these are common and normal physical responses to a traumatic event, and will often diminish with time.

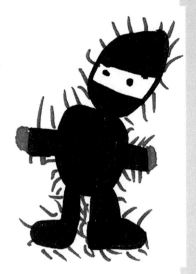

Because grieving requires a great deal of energy and stamina, grievers become susceptible to illnesses such as common colds and the flu. Headaches, stomach or gastrointestinal pains, skeletal aches, colds and sore throats can be grief-related. Some teens manifest sicknesses similar to the ones experienced by the person who died, as they unconsciously process their grief. Illness is sometimes the body's unconscious expression of the tensions and stresses of grief. Symptoms should not be minimized, nor should one assume that they are only caused by grief. If symptoms persist, medical treatment, in addition to grief counseling or a peer support group, may be important for a teen's physical and psychological health. Communicating and talking in a safe environment often helps alleviate both the physical and emotional pain of the griever.

Playing

Teens often process their grief through play. Play activities express grief in unique ways often unrecognized by adults who see play as "just fun," inappropriate or disrespectful. Playing and toys—the tools of play—can be creative, nonverbal expressions of grief thoughts, feelings and emotions. Engaging in sports, board and video games, table games, movies, and hobbies and collections might be effective ways for teens to grieve. Sometimes, adults are skeptical or critical of teens' play. These judgments do not support teens who are processing their grief. Play is a very appropriate, healthy and effective way for teens to grieve.

"My dad doesn't really understand that when I play air hockey it helps me get some of my feelings out. Not everybody wants to talk about how they feel. I don't. He thinks I don't care about what happened to my mom."

—Jake, 15

Regressive Behaviors

Regression—reverting to younger behaviors—is a common reaction to loss when a young person feels insecure or uncertain. Regression may be demonstrated in various behaviors, including:

- clinging to people
- clumsiness
- timidity
- thumb-sucking, bed-wetting
- stuttering or other speech changes
- immature play

Helpful Hints about Regression

Some teens feel extremely anxious about the future, wanting to hold tightly to the security of the past and the surviving adult. Regressive behaviors are ways of coping with the death and its radical changes. These behaviors often go away as the intense grieving eases. If behaviors persist, a medical evaluation and/or counseling may be needed.

Struggling with Core Belief Systems

Teens often experience a death as a direct, personal insult to their own belief system. They want to believe in an orderly, just world in which only elderly people die and young people thrive. This order is disrupted by an untimely, unexpected death. "Death happens in other people's worlds, but not mine," is the belief of many teens. Suddenly, disorder and unfairness strike, questioning all previously considered values and systems related to the meaning of life.

Adolescence is a time of reexamining, critiquing and investigating alternative world views and belief systems. A death often propels a teen to question previously held spiritual values and religious beliefs.

Some teens become intensely invested in spiritual and religious pursuits as an expression and release for their grieving. Other teens become resistant and even turn against anyone or anything connected to spirituality or religion.

Many teens attempt to find their own explanation for the death. Wondering about the afterlife and pondering the eternal destiny of the deceased is a common spiritual and mental pursuit for grievers. Expect and allow them to find their own answers.

"I think a lot about my mom, wondering if she's in heaven or hell."

—Sharon, 15

Suicidal Talk or Behavior

It is not unusual for teens to express verbally, or in writing, that they would like to join the person who died, or that they wish that they were dead. It is important to note that all references to suicide and suicidal behaviors should be taken seriously.

Helpful Hints about Suicidal Talk or Behavior

The young person should be asked directly if he or she has thoughts or plans to take his or her own life. Not all young people who talk about suicide act on it, but most who complete suicide have talked about it with someone. It is advisable to err on the side of caution and seek professional help for an evaluation and appropriate intervention.

Some of the warning signs indicating the need for professional help or evaluation for suicidal risk include:

- continuous or persistent talk about wanting to join the deceased
- increased reckless behaviors
- a sudden change in attention to appearance
- giving away possessions
- talking about wanting to die, especially with details of how
- withdrawal from friends and prolonged depression
- abuse of substances

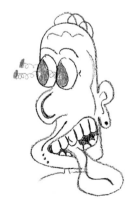

Unexplainable Sounds, Sightings and Smells

Many young people experience sounds, visions and smells related to the person who died or circumstances of the death. They tend to talk about these experiences only with trusted people whom they believe will understand and accept them. Examples of this, experienced by teens at The Dougy Center, include:

Gail, 15:

"My sister had her leg amputated when she was nine years old because of cancer. She had this false leg and foot that sounded heavy on the stairs. Since she died, I've heard that sound on the stairs a few times when I was home alone. I wasn't frightened or anything; I just went to the stairs and started talking to her. I think it's sort of neat to think she was there with me."

Jenni, 18:

"I've had these weird sightings of my mom. This ghosty-green cloud moved through my apartment a few times. At first I was scared, but I decided it was my mom checking up on me. My mom was always interested in what was happening with me. She wasn't nosy or controlling, just sort of amused and interested. So I bet anything she's still coming by now and then to see me."

Chad, 19:

"I was walking through the mall and saw this guy. I knew he was my dad. He was walking through the crowd. His head and hat looked exactly like my dad. He walked like my dad. The coat he wore was exactly like my dad's, with a dark blotch on the back. I was sort of in a daze as I hurried to catch up with him. I got almost up to him, when he suddenly turned around. I was shocked when it wasn't my dad's face. I almost tripped trying to change directions. I felt so embarrassed. Then I really felt stupid and angry at myself for thinking a dead person would come back."

Karen, 16:

"My dad smoked a pipe. More than once I've smelled the smoke from his pipe go through our house. My mom says that she has smelled it, too."

Helpful Hints about Sensory Experiences

Although experiences of seeing, smelling or hearing the deceased may seem unusual or strange to the teen or to others, they are actually very common. Unless the teen is experiencing destructive or disturbing behavior patterns or troubling behavior, don't be overly concerned about reports of unexplainable sounds, sightings or smells.

Basic Needs of Grieving Teens and How You Can Help

Assurances

Grieving teens want to feel certain that their parent or caregiver is healthy, balanced and in control. Parents should feel free to express emotions, but need to find adult support rather than depend upon the teen for support.

Boundaries

Young grievers need to know that adults care enough to set loving, specific limitations on their behavior. Reasonable and consistent boundaries provide safety and support teens during a period of disorienting change.

Choices

Teens are empowered when they are given choices and options. In the face of death, they often feel powerless and out of control. Providing the teen with informed choices and accepting his or her decisions can help him or her regain a sense of balance, and show that you respect their decision-making abilities.

Food

Grief work uses and depletes energy. Healthy, nutritious food provides fuel, so have it available in large quantities. Plan eating times that are comfortable and relaxed.

Listeners

Private grieving becomes public mourning when a teen finds an accepting listener in whom to confide. A safe listener can have a profound influence on the life of a young person who is grieving.

Models

Teens watch the adults in their lives to learn how (or how not) to grieve and mourn. Adults who abuse alcohol or other drugs, who refuse to display any emotions, or who run from their grief in other ways are poor models for a healthy grief process. Adults who share their own private grieving and mourning can be constructive role models.

Privacy

Much of grieving is a private process, including reflection, contemplation, communication, evaluation, emotion, determination and memorialization. Remember to respect the privacy of grieving teens.

Recreation

Grievers need time to have fun. Either with friends or alone, recreation can be a means of grieving or can provide a much needed break from the serious work of grieving.

Routines

Routines, such as regular bed times, meals and chores, provide a safe, predictable environment for teens. Routines allow teens consistency; they do not have to constantly worry about what will happen next.

Sleep

Grieving can cause fatigue. Grief work demands rest. Try to ensure that your teen gets enough sleep.

"I sleep more than I used to; but I'm still tired most of the time. Sleep feels so good. It is as if my bed has become my best friend."

—Carl, 18

Truth

Truth heals and promotes a healthy grieving process. Grievers appreciate truthful disclosure about all information relating to the person who died, the circumstances and potential changes that will affect them.

Water

Grievers often experience dehydration. Water is a forgotten healer. Caffeine dehydrates; water hydrates. Offer healthy liquids to teens who are grieving.

Funerals, Ceremonies and Memorialization

Being able to say "goodbye" in a significant way is important to grieving teens. Some teens feel cheated because there was no opportunity to have a significant "farewell" before the person died. Although face-to-face contact is no longer possible, you might invite the young person to think about creating a "farewell" ritual. Even after public ceremonies, teens can brainstorm about "farewell" rituals that might be meaningful for them. For example, you may invite teens to:

- write goodbye letters and read them at the grave, site of the ashes, and/or a special place
- light candles and share memories of the deceased
- spread the person's favorite fragrance on a favorite site and talk about the person
- creatively organize memories into scrapbooks, photo albums, videos and journals
- revisit places and/or create rituals of remembrance and respect at the place of the death, the grave site, the cremains site and other important places
- create art forms, such as paintings, collages or drawings
- write music, prose or poetry
- allow teens to express their grief privately or publicly
- remember the person on special days like their birthday and date of death

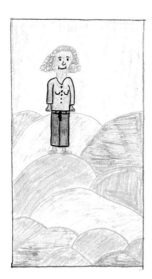

My Grandma was a beautiful woman. She was a person who loved the countary side.

"Momories" is Kevin's poetic expression in tribute of his mother on Mother's Day. Kevin, 14, intended to entitle his poem Memories, but realized his typing error expressed his intention to memorialize his mother.

Momories

Memories of loving
Memories of ones who care,

Facing the forgotten,
Facing the ones who were always there.

Death is for the people,
For the ones who really care,

Life is for the living,
For the people who are strong and are here.

The world will never be the same,
I wish this could of all been just a dream.

The memories of ones who used to be here,
A memory of someone who used to be there,
Of a loved one who once and will always be there.

"My dad always invites me to go with him to my mother's favorite lake where we spread her ashes. Sometimes we light candles in the canoe or spread her favorite flowers. One time we took bottles of her perfume and put drops in the water. I really feel close to her and my dad."

—George, 16

Reminiscing about the past and the relationship with the deceased is a powerful tool for healing. Holidays, the anniversary of the death, the birthday of the deceased and other special days associated with the deceased are particularly important to remember and commemorate with existing or new rituals.

In preparation for a ritual or farewell ceremony, it is important to honor teens' needs for privacy and time alone. Teens will often participate in a remembrance ritual if they know that they will not be on display in front of adults or siblings. Choices about if and how they will participate in an event are also essential. Parents or caregivers who provide the impetus for rituals by providing creative ideas, transportation, the necessary funds and a teen's favorite food before or after the event will probably help the teen experience a meaningful "goodbye" ritual.

Always remember that an invitation for a ritual event turned down today doesn't mean that the invitation will always be turned down.

"My mom made me go with her and my brothers to Dad's grave. It sucked. We just stood around with her crying. I felt so stupid. As soon as I get my license, the first thing I'm going to do is to go to the grave by myself. I don't want to go up there with anyone else."

—Kelly, 13

Memorialization

Teens are very much aware of the traditional or transitional events at which the deceased will be absent, such as graduation, marriage and holidays. Transitional events are difficult for grieving teens and are often accompanied by waves of emotion. Specifically, transition times trigger thoughts about what life would have been like if the person had not died. Even years after the death, the teen is thinking, "If only my dad hadn't died, he would walk me down the aisle." Or, "If mom were here, she would help me put on this wedding dress." The thoughts of "if only" are boundless, and the grief erupts unexpectedly. Here are some ways you might help teens through transitional times:

- Invite the teen to participate in creating a ceremony remembering the deceased for an upcoming traditional or transitional event. Preparing the teen for the possibility that upcoming events, like holidays and anniversaries, may stir up feelings helps remove the surprise of the intensity of emotion.

- Explore some of the following questions and issues with your teen in regards to the upcoming holiday, anniversary or event:

1. How do we want to remember the person who has died?
2. How do you think he or she would like to be remembered at this time?
3. What would it be like for you if he or she were here?

Holidays

Special times of the year, such as Christmas and Thanksgiving, may also trigger emotions and memories for teens. On these occasions, teens may:

- experience more intense grief reactions than usual
- feel emotionally raw and confused by their reactions
- find it difficult to attend family and social events
- experience deep sadness and discouragement, accompanied by explosive anger and irritation
- conclude that not celebrating the holiday might reduce the emotional intensity
- refuse to attend a family celebration to keep from embarrassing themselves or being embarrassed by the emotional outbursts of others
- develop expectations that often are unmatched by realities
- magnify the absence of the deceased and life changes
- escalate "If only…" thinking and regrets about what they might have done differently

Helpful Hints about Holidays

Remind the teen that nothing can bring back the person who died, or that life is as it was on previous holidays. Also emphasize the reality that the young person is beginning a life that will not be shared or experienced by the deceased.

Keep in mind that the teen's mind is working on important issues which he or she may not be consciously aware of and cannot express. Holidays trigger fleeting thoughts and emotions that have been blocked because of preoccupation with routine school, sports and social activities. Thoughts of the holidays and other significant events highlight the reality of life without the significant person.

Many of the newly grieved teens agreed with Eric's critique (following page) of the upcoming holiday. Teens who had experienced at least one holiday since the death were more optimistic about the celebrations and talked about finding meaning in the holidays.

A teen at The Dougy Center asked his group of peers: "Does anyone else in here feel that Chistmas is going to be a big pain? This may be a stupid question, but I think my sister's death is going to make Christmas horrible for my parents and me! I just wish we could be done with it this year. I really wish we didn't have to have it."

—Eric, 13

Families at The Dougy Center have found that planning ahead for these events is helpful. One family planned a Christmas Eve event where, early in the evening, everyone was invited to the living room. They had set up a large, lit candle surrounded by many small, unlit candles. People were invited to share a memory about the person who died that summer. Some people chose not to light a candle or share, but many people did share, including preschool children and teenagers. The special ceremony allowed the participants to release emotions through some crying and a great deal of laughing. Everyone thanked the host for planning such a lovely memorial for the deceased.

Another family planned to visit the grave of the deceased, placing stones on the grave marker the day before Hanukkah. A different family chose to honor a relative in the mountains, by visiting the place where the person had died.

Inviting teens to suggest what types of ceremonies and rituals they might want and allowing them to be significantly involved in the holiday planning helps relieve anxieties and negative feelings they may have about upcoming holiday events. These rituals can also be planned for the anniversary of the death. Remember that some teens may choose not to participate in holiday or anniversary-of-death activities. We suggest allowing them to choose for themselves the manner and extent to which they participate in these events.

How Different Types of Deaths Impact Teens

The Death of a Friend

Peer relationships frequently seem more important to teens than family relationships. Therefore, the death of a friend may significantly affect young people in ways parents and other adults may not understand.

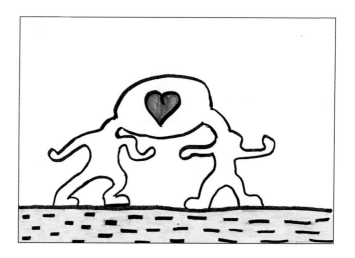

The death of a friend whom the parent never or seldom met may have little effect on the parent, but a huge impact on the teen. An adult who dismisses the impact of the teen's grief compounds strife with the teen and complicates the grieving process of the young person.

Following her boyfriend's death, Amy, age 17, angrily commented, "My parents act like his death shouldn't affect me this way. Somehow they just don't understand who he was to me. We really loved each other. We could talk about everything. Maybe if my parents had taken the time to get to know him. NO! They didn't want us together. I guess they'll never understand."

When a peer dies, teens are confronted with the realities of death, the possibilities of their own mortality and feelings of being abandoned by close friends. Young people often believe that they are immune to death. They think that death only happens to old people. When a friend dies, their entire world and beliefs are shaken to the core.

Often, teen friendships are up-and-down, on-and-off relationships. Grief complicates all relationships and ends up pulling people together or apart. After the death of a friend, some teens draw together to share their grief, while others are embarrassed and have difficulty sharing emotionally charged grief. It is common for teen friendships to revolve around fun. Grieving is not fun. The grief that follows the death of a peer is compounded by the added loss of peer friendships and fun times.

Trust is built with teens by telling them the truth about how, when and where a peer died. Secrecy, deception, half-truths and lies, even when intended to protect, will often backfire, creating a wedge of suspicion and anger. Teens need to know the truth and should be trusted with the truth. Teens want their questions answered with the complete truth. If you don't know the facts, then "I don't know" is the truth.

"They treated me like a stupid kid. I could tell they weren't telling me everything. They said it was an accident. I knew it was bigger. Why couldn't they say, 'It was suicide,' and tell me the truth?"

—Heather, 14

The Death of a Parent

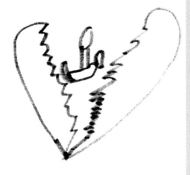

The death of a parent is usually a devastating, distressing experience in the life of a teen. When a parent dies, a young person's sense of security and stability in the world is turned upside down, regardless of the nature of the parent-child relationship. A parent's death disrupts the teen's life with radical complications. Suddenly, the teen is different from peers and feels strange and alone. The death of a parent becomes the defining event in the teen's life. A teen begins to define his life in two categories: "before" and "after" the death.

Statistics released by the 1995 U.S. Census Bureau indicate that nearly one million American children and teens under the age of 18 live with a widowed mother or father. More than 1% of young people under age 18 have experienced the death of their mother or father. Often, teens have difficulty talking to peers about a parent's death because they feel embarrassed about their emotions. They fear that they will cry or not be able to talk, and believe their friends won't understand. "I haven't even talked to my friends about my dad's death," is a common statement.

Some teens have conflictual, even abusive, relationships with parents and experience a sense of relief, ambivalence, guilt or regret after a parent dies.

33

parent dies. An abusive or neglectful relationship compounds the distress because the death means the loss of hope and opportunities for restoring the relationship.

Often, financial and daily living circumstances change radically when a parent dies, increasing the teen's feelings of loss of control and instability. Teens may have concerns about immediate physical and financial security. A parent or other adult can help by discussing the family's financial status, decisions and plans for the future with them. Telling the truth and giving choices will assist grieving teens to regain a sense of control of their lives.

Grieving teens are also coping with the realization that they will not have a father or mother to celebrate rites of passage—graduations, honors, marriage, childbirth and other future events. You can help them by recognizing that those events will be difficult times without the parent. As those events approach, it is important to help teens consider creative ways to memorialize the deceased. Some teens like to discuss how the deceased parent might have responded to their latest adventure, decision or problem.

After the death of a parent, teens can also experience strong grief reactions that are triggered by all kinds of events or circumstances. Here are some common triggers:

- Hearing the word "mother" or "father"
- Completing application forms that ask for parent information
- Father's Day or Mother's Day
- Peers' complaints about fathers or mothers
- The deceased's empty seat at the table
- Role changes around the house
- Anniversary dates, birthdays and holidays
- Smells associated with the person, e.g., perfumes, aftershave, pipe smoke, etc.
- Seeing someone who looks or walks like the deceased
- Hearing a song or favorite phrase of the deceased parent

"One of the things I hate to think about is that my dad won't be there for stuff that matters. He won't be at my graduations, my big dances, my wedding, the births of my babies. Wow, he'll never meet my husband or be my kid's grandpa."

—*Jamie, 17*

The death of a parent means the beginning of new life with a vulnerable, grieving parent, even if the parents were divorced. Teens tend to be astute caregivers of surviving parents. The teen left with only one biological parent is often also concerned, consciously or unconsciously, with the possible death of the surviving parent. Some teens neglect their own lives and interests to maintain harmony and consistency in the family. Other teens flee from home to stay away from the grieving parent's overprotectiveness and unrealistic role expectations.

Teens need to know that their surviving parent will continue to be a stable parent and will responsibly deal with the pain of losing a family member. Adolescents don't necessarily want to hear the full details about a parent's grieving, but want to feel secure that the parent is stable, functioning and finding help from peers or professionals.

"I stopped seeing my friends, wore my mom's clothes and started cooking. I kept trying to keep her here. I tried to be a 'super mom' to my little brother and sister."

—*Allie, 17*

The Death of a Sibling

The death of a brother or sister is significantly different from the death of a parent or another adult caregiver. Siblings are peers and experience a unique attachment as children of the same parents. Often, siblings hold confidences for each other from the parents. Suddenly, in many families the surviving child is "an only child" in a complex way that requires an unwanted adjustment of roles and relationships.

"I try to avoid my mom. She wants me to be with her and my little sister because she's scared. I just get up early and leave and don't come home until late. We always fight. It's best if I get out."

—*Danny, 19*

When a sibling dies, the grieving process might be complicated because of previous sibling conflicts and rivalries. The surviving brothers and sisters may feel intense guilt or regret about actions or things they said. The sibling may focus on the difficult times of conflicts, tensions and misunderstandings and feel stuck about resolving some of these memories and regrets.

You can help by providing opportunities for the teen to express those thoughts and emotions without judgment. Assisting the remorseful teen to find creative ways of reaching out to the deceased for forgiveness and reconciliation can bring a healing renewal and new equilibrium.

"Who will remember my childhood with me? We shared so many adventures together when no one else was there. We played house, read in the attic, caught salamanders, stole candy, and played doctor. No one will remember and laugh with me."

—Maria, 14

Grieving parents need to find ways to balance their grief over the death of a child, with attention and focused involvement with surviving children who need to feel valued and accepted. A teen's resentment toward the deceased sibling may grow because of the inordinate amount of attention and value expressed for that child. The teen may think, "I need to die to get my parents' attention." Most grieving parents find attending to the life of the surviving children, as well as dealing with their child's death, a very difficult balancing act. Teens may be overlooked as needing nurturing and emotional support. Parents may also become overly protective, smothering the surviving teen.

"Everybody was so focused on my sister and her death and my parents, that I became invisible. Nobody even talked to me. My parents were wrapped up in their own fog. I was too big to be treated like a little kid, so everybody sort of forgot me."

—Tracy, 14

Siblings will grieve the death of a brother or sister in their own unique way. Permission to grieve according to their own individual needs will enhance the possibility of a healthy grieving process. Rigid expectations and demands will hinder the process and can also generate anger and frustration.

"I'm so sick of my mom insisting that I go to my sister's grave. It sucks. She always stands over it sobbing. My dad doesn't have to be there. She makes me feel so guilty. She needs to be there, but not me. I am beginning to hate my sister for dying and putting me through this crap."

—*Kelly, 13*

"Who am I?" is an ongoing question for the developing teen. A sibling death calls into question the teen's previous identity as a brother or sister, especially for those who are left as the only living child. A teen now asks, "Now that my sibling died, who am I? Am I still a brother or sister?"

When others ask questions about their family, the grieving teen might struggle with how to answer. Responding "I'm an only child" doesn't seem to accurately describe the situation, but "My sister died and I'm the only one left" may provoke responses the teen does not want to deal with. "I don't have any living brothers or sisters" may be more personal than the teen wants to reveal, but "I don't have any brothers or sisters" may feel like a betrayal of the deceased sibling. Helping the teen anticipate and plan for these questions may help prevent awkward and distressing situations.

Coping With Death Under Special Circumstances

A Violent Death

When teens experience a violent death, such as a murder, a drunken driving crash or other violent act that leads to death, their basic belief system is thrown into turmoil. Teens typically consider themselves and their families immune from such violent acts. Suddenly, their innocence and certainties are shattered and their world no longer feels safe. They question the foundation and purpose of life itself. Thoughts and feelings about the person who died and the person(s) who caused the death get all mixed up, and teens feel confused.

Family members are tormented by powerful feelings and thoughts about the deceased and the perpetrator. Revenge and animosity toward the perpetrator can get in the way of truly grieving for the person who died.

The social stigma of a violent death

People often harshly and unfairly judge the victims or their family members after a violent death. This helps people protect themselves from believing that someone they love could be murdered. People sometimes believe that the family of the murder victim must have, in some way, contributed to the event. They feel safer if they think that "bad things only happen to bad people." Obviously, this social attitude alienates those who are impacted by a homicide or violent death. Additionally, people often do not know what to say or how to support the surviving family, so they stay away, contributing to the family's feelings of isolation.

After my dad's funeral, my aunt told me that my dad would still be alive if he hadn't been so interested in guns and people with guns. My dad got shot by a robber with a gun. It wasn't my dad's gun. He was at the grocery store. My aunt is wrong."

—*Brian, 17*

Additional issues of coping after a homicide or violent death

After a violent death people's curiosity and questioning can be intrusive and irritating to many teens. The initial media exposure may be sensationalized, promoting conjectures or outright errors that are never retracted or corrected. These experiences can cause resentment toward police and media crews. Sound bites and video clips don't give a significant explanation of what happened. Anger, resentment, bitterness and frustration mount for the grieving teens, not only toward the perpetrator but toward others in the community who rush to conclusions based on incomplete, and often inaccurate, information.

Another factor that may make coping more difficult after a homicide is the impact of the ongoing legal investigation and, potentially, a trial. Family members are told by police not to discuss the case with anyone, which makes it difficult to get support.

which makes it difficult to get support. Sometimes a family member is a suspect, which adds intense stress on everyone. If the murderer is caught, there is someone to be angry with, but families seldom feel that justice has been done, no matter what the verdict is. Even if the accused is found guilty and sentenced to life in prison, that person gets to eat, breathe and sleep; the deceased doesn't. The reality is that no form of justice can return a loved one. If a suspect is never caught, many teens express fear that the person will come and harm them.

Anger, disappointment, rage and revenge toward the perpetrator, the police and/or the legal system continues to divert energy away from healing. Because of the time lag between the violent act and the verdict, many supportive persons move on with their own lives and are unable to support the family. Sometimes, victims feel alone, forgotten and isolated. Victims Assistance programs, peer groups for victims, clergy persons, family members and professional grief therapists can be of great assistance to the survivors.

Death by Suicide

The act of suicide produces an array of unwanted thoughts and feelings toward the person who died and about the circumstances under which the death occurred. "Why?" seems to be the foremost question for teens who have had someone die from suicide. Thoughts of unfulfilled promises, disrupted relationships, missed warning signs and haunting, unanswered questions relentlessly preoccupy the teen's mind. Real or imagined images of the final scene may persist and cause emotional turmoil.

Often, the teen finds no satisfying answers to very difficult questions. Because there is such a stigma associated with suicide, many people are unaware of current research findings that suggest chemical imbalances in the brain as a contributor to suicidal acts. As difficult to understand as it may be, for the suicidal person, taking his or her own life becomes the only possible act to get out of intense emotional pain. Helping teens understand that the suicidal person is not thinking clearly, or is suffering from a brain disease, may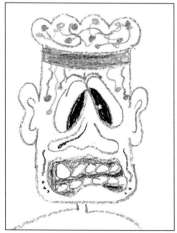
assist in their ability to process the meaning of this act.

Teens may be afraid that they are "fated" to die by suicide when a parent takes his or her own life. It is important to assist teens in under-standing and developing other ways to cope with life's inevitable disappointments and difficulties.

Some teens are relieved after a suicide because the person who died had been causing a great deal of tension and conflict in the family. Relief is a hard emotion to express or explain because it seems callous to feel that way. Although there is a sense of relief, teens can also feel guilty and become self-destructive and self-denigrating.

"Someone might ask about my dad. If I say he's dead, they might ask how he died. It is hard to tell them. I feel embarrassed; I just say he had heart failure."

—Cody, 11

Death from AIDS

It has been our experience that teens who have had a parent or sibling die of AIDS usually feel uncomfortable talking about the cause of death due to the social stigma associated with AIDS. Teens may fear that if they reveal that it was an AIDS-related death, they will be ostracized. Because young people in this situation tend to hold their feelings inside, they can experience a higher level of physical symptoms and concerns about their own health.

Don't force the teen to share the cause of death with others unless and until he or she is ready to do so. At the same time, allow the teen to talk about the person who died and to memorialize the deceased. Once the teen is ready to discuss the cause of death, you may want to help him or her gain a thorough understanding of AIDS and to think through how to respond when someone is critical about the disease. Finally, teens often benefit from participating in support groups with others who have experienced an AIDS death.

Death from Chronic Illness

When a family member's death is due to illness, teens sometimes develop fears around their own health, worrying that they, too, have the fatal disease or illness. After such a death, teens want to share common experiences of the dying process. They want to talk about things like hospitalization, medical procedures, emergencies, changes in personality due to an illness and how illness affects relationships.

Teens may also feel a sense of relief that the person died because the intense suffering and pain is over.

Accidental Death

Death from an accident often evokes fears involving lack of safety, loss of control, powerlessness and unpredictability. Accidental deaths may occur in a variety of circumstances, including car accidents, work-related injuries, sports-related accidents, etc. Teens need to share what they have been told about the accident and what they think actually happened.

When a Teen Witnesses a Death

Witnessing a scene where someone dies, or being threatened by a person or situation can result in stressful emotional and physical responses. It is especially traumatic for a teen to find the body after a murder or suicide. Being on the scene during emergency medical treatments can also be traumatizing. These incidents have dramatic effects on the mind and body of the young witness. Allowing the witness to express thoughts and feelings about the traumatic incident helps reduce its negative effects. Recounting the unfolding drama of the event and discussing the teen's own perceptions help the witness diminish the aftermath of the traumatic event. Repression and denial of thoughts and feelings associated with the trauma only serves to prolong the grieving process.

In some cases, young witnesses should see a professional for a crisis debriefing and evaluation. It is possible for teens to experience a delayed psychological and physical reaction to a horrific event. Without some intervention, a teen may develop a post-traumatic stress disorder. Although the reaction may be delayed, the symptoms of this disorder result in future complications to the teen's normal lifestyle. Delinquent behavior may be one expression of this disorder.

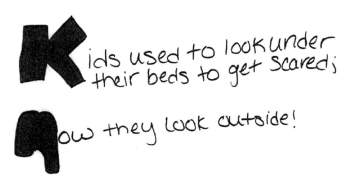

Kids used to look under their beds to get scared; now they look outside!

Witnessing a traumatic death can haunt the teen's thoughts. The death becomes the pivotal event around which everything else revolves for a long time. Life is defined as "before" and "after" the event, because their life has changed so dramatically. If the teen does not have healthy outlets for disturbing thoughts and feelings, he or she may seek relief in socially unacceptable ways, including addiction, shoplifting, obsessions and isolation.

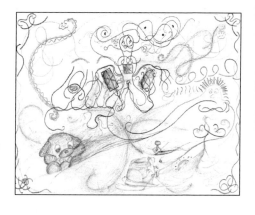

When Your Teen Needs Additional Help

It is important to assure young grievers that what they are going through is normal. Professional therapy is not necessary for many grieving teens. However, they do need the companionship and comfort of people who will listen and share and who have experience with, and are accepting of, their own grief issues and journeys.

Peer support groups for teens are often helpful. In groups, grieving teens can listen to and discuss their issues, fears and concerns in a safe, supportive environment. Peer support groups allow for frank expression and discussion about the deceased, the death and its circumstances. It is also a place to talk about the impact of the death, subsequent changes, relationships with family members and peers, strange experiences related to grief and a future faced without the deceased. Hearing the stories and grief journeys of peers and adults provides an opportunity for teens to:

- understand the nature of grief

- learn about alternative coping skills

- explore the adaptive methods of others

- normalize one's own experiences surrounding the death

The intensity of grieving and mourning should soften over time if the teen is making progress in the grief journey. Sometimes, certain grief reactions become prolonged and persistent, causing major life complications.

Here are some "red flag" behaviors that should be cause for concern and professional evaluation:

- Denying that the death occurred
- Panic, anxiety or fear which interferes with life
- Physical ailments that continue without identifiable medical causes
- Prolonged feelings of guilt or responsibility for the death
- Chronic depression
- Chronic anger or hostility
- Behavior that is reckless and life-endangering to self or others
- Prolonged changes in personality, personal appearance and/or behavior
- Consistent withdrawal from friends, family members, prior interests
- Prolonged changes in sleeping patterns
- Continuing problems with eating (overeating, under-eating, binging)
- Drug or alcohol abuse
- Sexual promiscuity
- Suicidal thoughts or actions

Be attentive to your own gut reactions when something is "not quite right" with the teen during his or her grieving process, and get help.

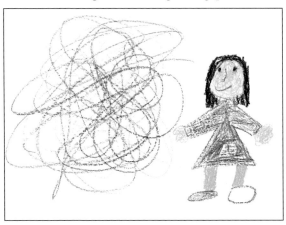

Seeking Professional Help

Because teens are focused on achieving independence and autonomy, they often have an innate resistance to accepting help. They may be especially reluctant to receive help from professionals, such as therapists, counselors, psychiatrists, clergy and doctors. The anxious, vulnerable teen is already struggling with normal issues and conflicts of adolescence, and the bereaved teen may feel stigmatized if professional help is needed.

Because being like their peers is of utmost importance, bereaved teens fear being classified as "different" or "weird."

"...children who lose a parent need two conditions to continue to thrive: a stable surviving parent or other caregiver to meet their emotional needs and the opportunity to release their feelings. Sheer physical care is not enough."

—Hope Edelman

Motherless Daughters, 1995

Teens are more likely to accept professional help if it is in the context of the entire grieving family—adults, children and teens. Inviting the teen to participate in therapy for the betterment of the family's situation is more likely to elicit a positive response than pointing out the teen's complicated grief signs as evidence of his or her need for counseling. It is also helpful to give teens informed options about therapy.

Tips for Parents

Grieving teens need parents and other adults who will take care of themselves and their own grief. Research indicates that caregivers are the primary bereavement models for teens. A teen is more likely to grieve in healthy ways when he or she has a supportive and healthy parent. Although parenting teen grievers is a difficult task for parents who are overwhelmed with their own bereavement, how a surviving parent copes with death has a major impact on their children.

Parents are also advised to be aware of the normal developmental changes that occur during adolescence. During the teen years, an emergent need for independence is addressed between the teen, parents and other adults. The ease of achieving independence and the degree of open conflict between the teen and his or her parents over independence issues are shaped by the parents' particular style of parenting.

"Since my mom's death, my dad is always checking up on me as if I were stupid. He's always interrogating me. He thinks I can plan out my life and give him a daily schedule."

—Scott, 17

"I don't want my mom's advice all the time. I can do it my own way. She is so controlling. I just wish she would leave me alone. No matter how I do it, I'm wrong. She criticizes everything. She's taken over my dad's way of dictating my life."

—Jeanna, 16

Some of the ways parents can be helpful to their teen during the grieving process include:

- listen, listen and listen before speaking
- act as a consultant to your teen: ask questions, listen to explanations and offer choices
- demonstrate that you trust yourself and your teen
- discuss important decisions and explain them to your teen
- problem solve together, considering many options
- negotiate reasonable limits
- build self-esteem by allowing your teen to experience the rewards and consequences of choices and behaviors
- offer advice and options if the teen wants to hear them
- empathize with your teen about the death, but make it clear that appropriate behavior is still expected
- avoid the temptation to overprotect your teens, or rescue them from the consequences of their behavior

"My mom told the police the truth after I shot out the windows in a vacant new home. When I bought the BB gun she said if I shot anything and got in trouble it was my trouble. I was mad at my dad's suicide, but I was mad at Mom for not lying to the neighbor for me. But now I know it was best for me."

—Casey, 14

How Teens Deal With a Parent Dating

Many parents who have had a spouse die experience less than enthusiastic responses from their teenagers when they begin to date. Welcome to the "My-Parent-Should-Not-Date Club," organized and supported by grieving teens and their younger siblings. Loyalty issues surface when the surviving parent begins to socialize or date. Teens may:

- be offended that their parent is being intimate with another person

- see friends and dates as enemies of the deceased spouse

- view the budding social life as a reminder that life will never return to its former reality

- resent the parent's friends, especially dates, as intrusions into a life that is already confused and disrupted

- become anxious about the possibility of a stepparent replacing the deceased parent

- resent that the potential stepsiblings may interfere with their relationship with their parent

- resent giving up special attention that a parent may have shown the teen after the death

Teens fear abandonment and displacement by the new significant other. In fact, a parent may already spend less time with and expend less energy on children than before the loss occurred. Young people also feel protective as they are aware of the potential hurt a parent will experience if a new relationship ends. A teen may feel threatened by loss of control and security as a parent's social life increases.

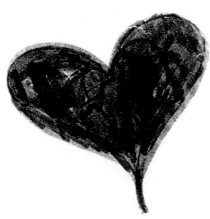

At The Dougy Center, teens often humorously, yet seriously, discuss the difficulties of having a dating parent. Just like anxious parents, they want to restrict the dating parent's activities with rules.

Here are a few guidelines they suggested:

Teen's Advice to a Dating Parent:

- Be home by midnight
- If you're going to be late, call
- I need to know the person(s) you're with
- I need to know where you're going and how to telephone you
- Don't get physical too soon
- Be sure you don't drink and drive
- Don't ride with someone who has been drinking
- Wear your seat belt. Sit only where there is a seat belt
- Go only to safe places
- Don't spring an engagement or wedding on me
- Listen to my concerns about your dates and dating
- Use birth control or, better yet, wait until marriage
- Be responsible

These rules sound familiar to any parent with teens. A parent who engages in open discussion about their own dating process will reduce the teen's anxieties and opposition.

Advice From Parents to Parents

Parents and caregivers of teens at The Dougy Center were asked, "If you had the opportunity to speak with other parents of newly bereaved teens, what would you say?" They responded:

Expect the unexpected. You'll be surprised by many of the reactions of your teen that don't meet your expectations.

Be an advocate for your teen at school or college. Consistently communicate with the administrators and teachers about the fact that your teen is grieving. Most people, including school personnel, have little experience with or knowledge about grieving teens and the grief process. People have limited experience with grief and often accept cultural myths about teen grief. You may have to educate them.

Don't expect your teen to grieve with you. Most teens talk very little to parents about their grieving. You probably will not be a primary person with whom they share.

Be aware that each teen is unique, therefore grieves uniquely.
Don't expect your children to grieve in the same way. Expect great variety.

♥

Recognize and respect the importance of a teen's privacy. Don't snoop, intrude into their space, or always be in their face. Teens may become more secretive and perhaps more prone to engage in detrimental behavior if they feel their privacy is being invaded.

♥

Appreciate a teen's unique pace and timing of grief. Your teen's process will be different from your own. Allow it, expect it and encourage it.

♥

Model grieving for and with your teen. It is important for your teen to know how you're doing. Explain what's going on for you and what you're doing to mourn and take care of your needs.

♥

Talk about the person who died in everyday conversations. Don't stop talking about the person as if he or she weren't in your lives. Talk about the deceased as a real person with a history, experiences, opinions, strengths and weaknesses.

♥

Allow your teen independence to grow and change. Resist the temptation to cling and hold onto the teen to meet your own needs. Encourage them to seek and fulfill their dreams and goals. Deal with your own grief issues around letting your teen go. Control will cause rebellion and resistance.

♥

Don't rely on the teen for too much support. You may feel unsafe or anxious without the young person's presence. Find your own peer support group or a grief counselor so your teen does not become your caregiver.

♥

Allow the teen to step outside his or her grief sometimes. Everyone needs some fun and escape from the pain. Fun and play is therapeutic and part of the grief process, too.

♥

Be aware that your teen may be protective of you. Your teen may be worried about you and want to take care of you. He or she may also be overprotective because of the fear of losing you, too.

Remember your teen's grief may erupt unexpectedly. An approaching anniversary, a big event, a news story, finding memorabilia or other grief stimuli may cause unexpected emotional outbursts.

♥

Establish and keep clear, specific communications with your teen. Discuss your plans, limitations, expectations and concerns. Talk and listen to your teen.

♥

Realize that your teen is thinking about a future that will not include the person who died. Who will walk me down the aisle? Who will I go hunting with this summer? Who will be the grandmother to my children? Who will remember our childhood secrets? These are difficult questions for your grieving teen.

♥

Don't try being both mother and father. It won't work. Don't try being a sister or brother either. Be yourself.

♥

Celebrate and create rituals of memory. In time, the family will learn to live with the pain and loss of the deceased person. But many teens are afraid that the person will be forgotten. It is important to find ways to share memories and retain a sense of the person's contribution to the family.

♥

Find help for yourself. Try friends, a peer support group, a clergy person and/or a grief therapist. Your healthy adaptation to life without the deceased person is the most important influence on your teen's ability to adapt and heal.

♥

Be available at the most inopportune times. Teens often are ready to talk late at night, early in the morning or times that don't coincide with your schedule or plans. Be available and seize those opportunities.

The Bill of Rights of Grieving Teens

A common topic raised by teens is their frustration with the lack of rights they have to grieve as teens. They feel that many adults strip them of rights that would benefit their grief process. At one of the teen groups at The Dougy Center, bereaved teens discussed a bill of rights for themselves. There was a great deal of discussing, arguing, rewording and compromising before the final draft was agreed upon. Here is their final draft.

A grieving teen has the right to...

Know the truth about the death, the deceased and the circumstances

Have questions answered honestly

Be heard with dignity and respect

Be silent and not tell you his or her grief emotions or thoughts

Not agree with your perceptions and conclusions

See the person who died and the place of the death

Grieve any way she or he wants without hurting self or others

Feel all the feelings and to think all the thoughts of his or her own unique grief

Not to have to follow the "Stages of Grief," as outlined in a high school health book

Grieve in one's own unique, individual way without censorship

Be angry at death, at the person who died, at God, at self and at others

Ignore people who are insensitive bigots who spout clichés

Have his or her own theological and philosophical beliefs about life and death

Be involved in the decisions about the rituals related to the death

Not be taken advantage of in this vulnerable mourning condition and circumstances

Have irrational guilt about how he or she could have intervened to stop the death

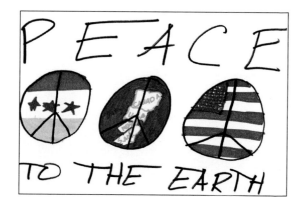

Resources

Also by The Dougy Center for Grieving Children

More in our Guidebook Series:

- **35 Ways to Help a Grieving Child**

If you know a child or teen who has experienced a death, this guidebook presents you with simple and practical suggestions for how to support him or her. Learn what behaviors and reactions to expect from grieving children at different ages, ways to create safe outlets for children to express their thoughts and feelings, and how to be supportive during special events such as the memorial service, anniversaries and holidays. Available in English and Spanish.

- **Helping Children Cope with Death**

This guidebook offers a comprehensive overview of how children grieve and strategies to support them. Based on The Dougy Center's work with thousands of grieving children and their families, you will learn how children understand death, how to talk with children about death at various developmental stages, how to be helpful, and when to seek outside help. This book is useful for parents, teachers, helping professionals and anyone trying to support a grieving child. Available in English and Spanish.

- **What About the Kids? Understanding Their Needs in Funeral Planning and Services**

This book addresses the best practices for funeral and memorial services with children and teens. Learn how to include children in these rituals and to involve them in the process. You will find suggestions from children and teens about what was helpful and unhelpful about the funeral or memorial service they attended.

- **Helping the Grieving Student: A Guide for Teachers**

At some point, every teacher will encounter a student who has been affected by a death. This guidebook is an essential resource for elementary, middle and high school teachers, offering practical tips and information on how to respond to a child or teen who has experienced a death in his or her family.

- **When Death Impacts Your School: A Guide for School Administrators**
A valuable resource for school personnel who are faced with a death or tragedy in their school community, this guidebook includes suggestions for how schools can help students—by addressing concerns, organizing memorials and offering support. It also includes instructions for developing a school intervention plan after a death, how to address issues related to suicide and violence, and how to decide when outside help is needed.

Activity Books:

- **After a Death: An Activity Book for Children**
With a mixture of creative activities and tips for dealing with changes at school, home and with friends, this is a helpful tool for all grieving children. It includes a variety of drawing and writing exercises to help children remember the person who died, and learn new ways to live with the loss. Available in English and Spanish.

- **After a Suicide Death: An Activity Book for Grieving Kids**
In this hands-on, interactive activity book, children who have had someone in their lives die of suicide can learn from other grieving kids. The workbook includes drawing activities, puzzles, stories, advice from other kids and helpful suggestions for navigating grief after a suicide death.

- **After a Murder: An Activity Book for Grieving Kids**
Through the stories, thoughts and feelings of other kids who have had someone in their lives murdered, this hands-on workbook allows children to see that they are not alone in their feelings and experiences. The workbook includes drawing activities, puzzles and word games to help explain confusing elements specific to a murder, such as the police, media and legal system.

- **Memories Matter: 70 Activities for Grieving Children & Teens**
Memories Matter features 70 activities to use with children and teens in peer support groups or for parents to use with their children. These activities are categorized by topic and are designed to help children process their unique grief.

DVDs:

- **Helping Teens Cope with Death**
(21 minutes) is a window into the lives of six grieving teens who attended peer support groups at The Dougy Center. The DVD and 12-page companion guide provide insight to the thoughts, feelings, and changes that teens often experience. The DVD and guide are a resource for training purposes, or for general viewing by teens, parents, therapists, counselors and others.

- **Understanding Suicide, Supporting Children**
(24 minutes) provides insight on the emotions and experiences that children, teens and families bereaved after a suicide death often go through, and offers ways to help. The DVD and 12-page companion guide are a resource for training purposes; for general viewing by children, teens, parents, therapists, counselors, professionals in the field of suicide prevention/postvention; and for anyone seeking to better understand suicide and how to support those grieving a suicide death.

- **Acting Out: The Scarlet D's on their Grief Trip**
This documentary (75 minutes), produced by American Lifeograph Productions and filmed by Lani Jo Leigh, chronicles The Dougy Center's first Teen Theatre Troupe, The Scarlet D's, as they create, direct, and perform an original production about their experiences with grief. The DVD also includes complete footage of the Troupe's live performance (45 minutes). An emotionally engaging video, this is a powerful tool for grief support programs, schools, community groups, and families.

The above resources can be ordered by calling 503-775-5683 or through The Dougy Center's website at **www.dougy.org.**

What is The Dougy Center?

The mission of The Dougy Center is to provide loving support in a safe place where children, teens and their families who are grieving a death can share their experiences as they move through their healing processes. Through our National Center for Grieving Children & Families, we also provide support and training locally, nationally and internationally to individuals and organizations seeking to assist children and teens in grief.

The Dougy Center serves children and teens, ages 3 to 18, and young adults, 18 to 30 and their families who have experienced the death of a parent or sibling (or, in our teen and young adult groups, a friend), to accident, illness, suicide or murder. Peer support groups are coordinated by professional staff and trained volunteers. In addition, the parents or caregivers of the youth participate in support groups to address their needs and the issues of raising children following a traumatic loss.

When The Dougy Center was established in 1982, it was the first grief peer support program of its kind in the country. In response to numerous requests for information about our program, The Dougy Center has developed trainings and publications to help other communities establish centers for grieving children and families. Through our National Center for Grieving Children, The Dougy Center has trained individuals and groups throughout the world and publishes a National Directory of Children's Grief Services, updated annually.

The Dougy Center is a 501(c)3 nonprofit organization and raises its entire budget through contributions from individuals, businesses and foundations. We receive no federal funding or third-party payments. Participating families may contribute to the program, but there is no fee for service. While families receiving services contribute what they can, many do not have the financial resources to donate. Because The Dougy Center never turns a family away because of their inability to contribute, we are completely reliant upon private support from our friends in the community.

How can I support The Dougy Center or get additional information about its programs?

Contributions to The Dougy Center are tax-deductible to the full extent allowable under IRS guidelines. Your gift can be made out to The Dougy Center and mailed to us at the address below.

You can also receive additional information about:

- other guidebooks available from The Dougy Center

- videos and other resource materials available from The Dougy Center

- training for developing a children's grief center in your area

- the National Summer Institute held annually at The Dougy Center on developing a children's grief center in your area

- how to schedule a training or presentation in your area

- supporting The Dougy Center and its local and national programs to assist grieving children through a will or bequest

Write, call, fax or email:

The Dougy Center
P.O. Box 86852
Portland, OR 97286

503-775-5683
Fax: 503-777-3097

Email: help@dougy.org
Website: www.dougy.org

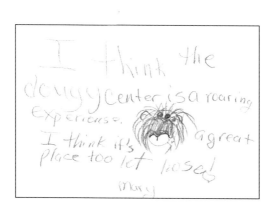

Contributors to the Guidebook comprise The Dougy Center staff:

Amy R. Barrett, M.S.
(former) Director of Children's Grief Services/Writing & Editing

Joan Schweizer Hoff, M.A.
Associate Director/Writing & Editing

Donna L. Schuurman, Ed.D.
Executive Director/Writing & Editing

Donald W. Spencer, M.Div., M.Ed., M.Coun.Psy.
(former) Director of Family Services/Editing

Inside Art:
Provided by teens from The Dougy Center

Design:
Fran Fitzsimon/Fitzsimon GRAFIX

Cover Design:
Deb Minkler

Copy Editor:
Stephanie W. Gray

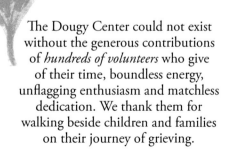

The Dougy Center could not exist
without the generous contributions
of *hundreds of volunteers* who give
of their time, boundless energy,
unflagging enthusiasm and matchless
dedication. We thank them for
walking beside children and families
on their journey of grieving.

Notes

Notes

80376935R00038

Made in the USA
San Bernardino, CA
26 June 2018